NOURISHMENT BLUE PRINT

Mastering the act of Nutritious Eating

Michael Rodger

1

INTRODUCTION

In the bustling tapestry of modern life, where fast food joints beckon from every corner and time seems to evaporate faster than water in the desert sun, the quest for a healthier lifestyle emerges as a beacon of hope. Welcome to the pages of "Culinary Renewal: Nourishing Body, Nurturing Soul," a captivating journey into the life of one individual's courageous endeavor to cultivate a healthy eating habit and transform their diet from a chaotic mishmash of convenience to a harmonious symphony of nourishment.

Imagine entering the world of our protagonist, Alex, whose story unfolds against the backdrop of a society perpetually on the go, and where nutritional novelties tantalize from every social media feed. As the dawn breaks on the first page, we find Alex standing at a crossroads. The reflection in the mirror whispers untold stories of late-night snacking and guilt-laden indulgences. Yet, amidst the chaos, a spark ignites—a desire for change, a yearning for vitality that transcends mere appearance.

The journey begins with a single step, as it often does. Armed with a determination as sturdy as a foundation stone, Alex confronts the pantry shelves once stocked with sugary cereals and processed snacks. In their place, a vibrant array of whole grains, crisp vegetables, and lean proteins emerge. The kitchen becomes a sanctuary, where pots and pans become instruments of transformation, and flavors merge to create symphonies of satisfaction.

The path is far from smooth, and early trials reveal the grip of old habits. The memory of a warm slice of pizza shared with friends lingers like a nostalgic melody, and the temptation of a sugary treat after a taxing day beckons like a siren's call. Yet, Alex stands strong, guided by newfound knowledge of the intricate dance between nutrients and well-being. Each day becomes a canvas, a chance to craft a masterpiece of health through choices made at the breakfast table, in the office cafeteria, and at the dinner plate.

As the seasons shift, the narrative unfolds like a budding flower, revealing layers of growth and self-discovery.

Alex's journey takes them from the farmer's market, where vibrant produce tells tales of the earth's bounty, to the serene haven of a meditation retreat, where mindful eating awakens a deeper connection to sustenance. Through the pages, we witness a metamorphosis—a metamorphosis not just of the body, but of the spirit.

The beauty of "Culinary Renewal" lies not only in the evolution of Alex's habits but in the universal truths it unveils. In a world often overshadowed by fads and quick fixes, the book speaks to the timeless wisdom of nourishing not just the body, but also the soul. As Alex explores the intricate balance of nutrients and flavors, they also encounter the delicate interplay of emotions and well-being.

As the final pages draw near, a sense of fulfillment permeates the air. Alex's journey, while deeply personal, resonates with every reader who has embarked on their own quest for vitality. The transformation, though prompted by the desire for healthier eating, touches upon the fundamental quest for self-discovery, self-love, and authenticity.

So, dear reader, as you delve into the pages of "Culinary Renewal: Nourishing Body, Nurturing Soul," prepare to be captivated not only by Alex's culinary escapades but by the tapestry of growth, resilience, and joy that emerges from their pursuit of healthier choices. In this world of endless distractions, let this book serve as a guiding light—an invitation to embrace change, to savor the journey, and to find nourishment not only in the food we eat but in the boundless potential that resides within us all.

Chapter 1

Nourishment

Nourishment is a fundamental aspect of human existence. It encompasses the sustenance of both the body and the mind. The multifaceted concept of nourishment extends far beyond mere food; it encompasses a rich tapestry of ideas, practices, and experiences that shape our physical, mental, and emotional well-being.

At its core, nourishment is the process by which living organisms receive the vital elements necessary for their growth, development, and survival. For humans, this primarily involves the consumption of food and water. Food, in its diverse forms, is the cornerstone of nourishment, providing the essential nutrients and energy required to fuel our daily activities.

The spectrum of nourishment is vast, encompassing a plethora of dietary preferences and traditions. Some opt for a plant-based diet, embracing fruits, vegetables, grains, and legumes as their primary sources of sustenance. Others prefer a more omnivorous approach, incorporating meat, dairy, and seafood into their meals. Each culinary path reflects not only cultural heritage but also personal beliefs and values.

Nourishment transcends the physical act of eating. It extends into the realm of culinary arts, where food becomes an expression of creativity and culture. Talented chefs craft dishes that tantalize the senses, combining flavors, textures, and aesthetics to create culinary masterpieces. Food, in this context, becomes an art form, nourishing not just the body but also the soul.

Beyond the plate, the act of sharing a meal with loved ones fosters a sense of connection and belonging. Family gatherings, holiday feasts, and intimate dinners with friends are all occasions where nourishment takes on a communal dimension. Conversation flows as freely as wine, strengthening bonds and nourishing the human need for social interaction.

Nourishment isn't solely about the quantity of food consumed but also the quality. The modern world offers a plethora of choices, from fast food loaded with empty calories to organic, locally-sourced produce bursting with nutrients. Making informed choices about what we eat plays a pivotal role in maintaining good health.

The concept of mindful eating encourages individuals to savor each bite, appreciating the flavors and textures that nourish the palate. This practice not only enhances the dining experience but also fosters a deeper connection with one's body and its nutritional needs.

Nourishment isn't confined to the realm of physical health. It extends to mental and emotional well-being as well. Mental nourishment involves feeding the mind with knowledge, creativity, and stimulation. Engaging in lifelong learning, pursuing hobbies, and practicing mindfulness are all ways to nourish the intellect.

Emotional nourishment encompasses the nurturing of our feelings and relationships. Expressing emotions, seeking support when needed, and cultivating self-compassion are integral to emotional well-being. Like a well-balanced diet, emotional nourishment ensures a robust and resilient inner world.

Nature itself provides a source of profound nourishment. The great outdoors offers solace and rejuvenation, replenishing the spirit with its beauty and serenity. Time spent in nature, whether hiking through a forest, lounging on a beach, or simply gazing at the stars, nourishes the soul and provides a reprieve from the stresses of modern life.

Spiritual nourishment delves into the realm of faith and belief. For some, attending religious services and engaging in rituals provide a deep sense of spiritual sustenance. Others find spiritual nourishment through meditation, yoga, or the exploration of philosophical questions that give life meaning and purpose.

Nourishment is an evolving concept, adapting to the changing needs and desires of individuals and societies. In today's fast-paced world, convenience foods and digital distractions can hinder our ability to nourish ourselves holistically. Finding a balance between the convenience of modern life and the timeless principles of nourishment is an ongoing challenge.

In conclusion, nourishment is a rich and multifaceted concept that encompasses the sustenance of the body, mind, and spirit. It encompasses the choices we make about what we eat, how we eat, and how we nurture our intellectual, emotional, and spiritual well-being. To truly thrive, we must recognize the importance of nourishment in all its dimensions and strive to nourish ourselves and those around us in meaningful and sustainable ways

Ways of getting Nourishment

They are so many ways one can get nourished and they include

- Take healthy balance diet to nourish your body.
- Try a new vegetable or fruit every week.
- Cook a homemade soup from scratch.
- Enjoy a colorful salad with various vegetables.
- Savor a piece of dark chocolate for antioxidants.
- Take a multivitamin if your diet lacks nutrients.
- Try herbal teas for relaxation and health benefits.
- Make a smoothie with spinach, banana, and almond milk.
- Incorporate fermented foods like yogurt or kimchi.
- Plan and prepare meals ahead for the week.
- Practice portion control to avoid overeating.
- Take some walk to aid digestion
- Choose lean protein sources like poultry or tofu.
- Enjoy a bowl of oatmeal with nuts and berries.
- Have a small, healthy snack between meals.

- Cook with olive oil for its heart-healthy fats.
- Consume whole grains like quinoa or brown rice.
- Bake or grill foods instead of frying.
- Eat mindfully, savoring each bite.
- Experiment with plant-based protein sources.
- Go for cooking classes to learn and develop new cooking skills
- Grow your own herbs and vegetables.
- Share a meal with friends or family.
- Try intermittent fasting for metabolic benefits.
- Take a cooking challenge with unique ingredients.
- Reduce added sugar in your diet.
- Practice deep breathing to reduce stress.
- Eat foods rich in omega-3 fatty acids.
- Prioritize sleep for overall well-being.
- Practice gratitude to nourish your mental health.
- Enjoy a picnic in nature.
- Learn about your food's nutritional value.
- Attend a wellness retreat for relaxation.
- Cook a cultural dish from another country.
- Join a community garden for fresh produce.
- Take a nutrition course for knowledge.

- Share a homemade meal with a neighbor.
- Try a new type of cuisine you've never had.
- Volunteer at a local food bank.
- Practice mindful eating meditation.
- Engage in regular physical activity.
- Create a meal plan for variety.
- Enjoy a hot cup of green tea.
- Support local farmers' markets.
- Cook with fresh herbs like basil and cilantro.
- Learn about portion sizes for better control.
- Bake whole-grain bread at home.
- Make a fruit smoothie bowl for breakfast.
- Learn to read food labels for healthier choices.
- Share your favorite recipes with friends.
- Reduce processed food consumption.
- Eat a variety of nuts for different nutrients.
- Cook a hearty soup for a cozy meal.
- Practice yoga for flexibility and relaxation.
- Have a balanced meal before a workout.
- Make homemade salad dressings.
- Support sustainable food practices.
- Attend a food and wine pairing event.

- Try a new type of seafood.
- Create a garden in your backyard.
- Explore different cooking techniques.
- Consume foods high in fiber for digestion.
- Go for a hike in nature.
- Plan themed dinner nights with friends.
- Cook a dish from your cultural heritage.
- Take a break from screens during meals.
- Try intermittent fasting for metabolic benefits.
- Eat seasonally for fresher produce.
- Cook a stir-fry with colorful veggies.
- Visit a nutritionist for personalized advice.
- Learn about food allergies and sensitivities.
- Enjoy a glass of red wine in moderation.
- Explore the world of superfoods.
- Share a meal with someone you love.
- Practice mindfulness while grocery shopping.
- Start a food journal to track your choices.
- Make homemade popsicles with fruit juice.
- Cook with lean cuts of meat.
- Organize a healthy potluck with friends.
- Create a visually appealing meal presentation.

- Volunteer at a soup kitchen.
- Plan a picnic in the park.
- Cook with whole, unprocessed foods.
- Explore Asian cuisine with sushi or tofu dishes.
- Share recipes on social media for inspiration.
- Try a Mediterranean diet for heart health.
- Host a themed dinner party.
- Cook with seasonal herbs like sage or rosemary.
- Experiment with exotic fruits.
- Reduce food waste by using leftovers creatively.
- Practice portion control when dining out.
- Create a garden of edible flowers.
- Try a fruit you've never tasted before.
- Learn food preservation techniques like canning.
- Cook a one-pot meal for convenience.
- Explore Middle Eastern cuisine with hummus and falafel.
- Eat slowly to aid digestion.
- Take a cooking class online.
- Make your own energy bars.
- Share your cooking skills with a local community group.

- Try a high-protein diet for muscle health.
- Bake your own granola.
- Experiment with different salad greens.
- Join a cooking club for social cooking.
- Incorporate more leafy greens into your diet.
- Explore cooking with edible insects.
- Make a fruit-infused water for hydration.
- Learn about the benefits of probiotics.
- Cook a plant-based burger.
- Try a low-carb diet for weight management.
- Share a meal with a colleague.
- Cook with whole wheat pasta.
- Explore the world of cooking with herbs.
- Create a healthy meal prep routine.
- Attend a food festival in your city.
- Try a ketogenic diet for metabolic changes.
- Make your own salad dressing with olive oil.
- Experiment with different cooking oil
- Cook a dish with seasonal berries.
- Try a gluten-free diet for dietary needs.
- Make your own yogurt at home.
- Explore the benefits of intermittent fasting.

- Share a meal with a senior citizen.
- Cook a dish using ancient grains.
- Try a paleo diet for whole foods.
- Create a food-themed art project.
- Host a cooking competition with friends.
- Experiment with spiralized vegetables.
- Learn about food preservation methods.
- Try a low-sugar diet for better health.
- Make your own nut butter.
- Cook a dish with edible seaweed.
- Explore the benefits of a raw food diet.
- Host a healthy cooking workshop.
- Try a high-fiber diet for digestive health.
- Make your own pickled vegetables.
- Experiment with plant-based protein sources.
- Share a meal with a local farmer.
- Cook a dish using ancient grains.
- Try a paleo diet for whole foods.
- Create a food-themed art project.

Importance of Nourishment

Nourishment: The Cornerstone of Health and Well-being

In a world where information about diets, supplements, and miracle foods inundates us daily, it's easy to lose sight of a fundamental truth: nourishment is the cornerstone of health and well-being. While it's true that trends and fads in the realm of nutrition come and go, the importance of providing our bodies with the right nutrients remains constant. In this essay, we will explore the multifaceted significance of nourishment, from its role in physical health to its impact on mental and emotional well-being.

1. Physical Health:

Nourishing our bodies with the right balance of nutrients is essential for maintaining physical health. Our bodies are intricate machines that require a variety of vitamins, minerals, carbohydrates, proteins, and fats to function optimally. These nutrients are the fuel that powers every bodily process, from the beating of our hearts to the firing of neurons in our brains.

A well-balanced diet provides the vitamins and minerals necessary for building strong bones, maintaining healthy skin, and supporting our immune system. For example, calcium and vitamin D are vital for bone health, while vitamin C boosts the immune system's ability to fight off infections.

Moreover, nourishment plays a crucial role in preventing chronic diseases. A diet rich in fruits, vegetables, whole grains, and lean proteins can reduce the risk of heart disease, diabetes, and certain types of cancer. On the other hand, a diet high in processed foods, saturated fats, and added sugars can increase the risk of these conditions.

2. Cognitive Function:

Nourishment isn't limited to the body; it profoundly affects our cognitive function and mental clarity. The brain, although a small organ, consumes a significant portion of the body's energy and nutrients. Therefore, what we eat directly impacts our cognitive abilities.

Omega-3 fatty acids found in fish, nuts, and seeds have been linked to improved memory and cognitive function. Antioxidant-rich foods like berries and leafy greens help protect brain cells from damage caused by free radicals. B vitamins, found in whole grains, beans, and leafy greens, play a crucial role in neurotransmitter production, which affects mood and cognitive function.

Conversely, a diet high in sugar and processed foods has been associated with cognitive decline and an increased risk of neurodegenerative diseases like Alzheimer's. In essence, our brains thrive on nourishment just as much as our bodies do.

3. Energy and Vitality:

Consider nourishment as the fuel that powers your daily activities. The quality of that fuel greatly influences your energy levels and vitality. A diet filled with nutrient-dense foods provides sustained energy throughout the day, helping you stay active and alert.

Carbohydrates, in the form of whole grains, fruits, and vegetables, serve as the body's primary source of energy. They provide glucose, which is the fuel that powers our cells. Protein, found in foods like lean meats, beans, and dairy products, supports muscle growth and repair, ensuring we have the strength and vitality to perform daily tasks.

When our diet consists of empty calories from sugary snacks and beverages, we experience energy spikes followed by crashes. These fluctuations can lead to fatigue, mood swings, and a decreased ability to concentrate. Thus, nourishing our bodies with the right foods is crucial for maintaining consistent energy levels and vitality.

4. Emotional Well-being:

The connection between nourishment and emotional well-being cannot be overstated. The foods we eat have a direct impact on our mood and emotions. Consider how you feel after a heavy, greasy meal compared to a light, balanced one. Food can influence our emotions in various ways:

a. Serotonin Production: Certain foods, like those rich in tryptophan (an amino acid), can boost serotonin production in the brain. Therefore, a diet that supports serotonin production can help improve mood and reduce symptoms of depression.

b. Blood Sugar Regulation: The foods we eat affect our blood sugar levels. Rapid fluctuations in blood sugar can lead to irritability and mood swings. A diet that helps stabilize blood sugar, such as one high in complex carbohydrates and fiber, can promote emotional stability.

c. Gut-Brain Connection: Emerging research has highlighted the gut-brain connection, suggesting that the health of our gut microbiome influences our mood and mental health. Probiotic-rich foods like yogurt and fermented foods can support a healthy gut, potentially benefiting emotional well-being.

In conclusion, nourishment is not just about filling our stomachs; it's about providing our bodies and minds with the essential elements they need to thrive. From physical health and cognitive function to emotional well-being and vitality, the importance of nourishment cannot be overstated. It's a lifelong investment in our health and happiness, and making informed choices about what we eat is one of the most significant steps we can take towards a better, more fulfilling life. So, let's savor the opportunity to nourish ourselves and, in doing so, unlock our full potential

Cultivating a Healthy Eating Habit

<u>Chapter 2</u>

Set Clear Goal on Your Diet

Setting clear goals when it comes to healthy eating habits is essential for achieving and maintaining overall well-being. Well-defined goals provide direction, motivation, and a sense of accomplishment. Here's a comprehensive overview of the importance and steps to set clear goals for healthy eating habits:

Importance of Setting Clear Goals

Clarity: Clear goals help you understand what you're working towards, preventing confusion and uncertainty.

Motivation: Goals provide a reason to make positive changes and stick to them, especially when faced with temptations.

Focus: Having specific goals helps you concentrate on what's important, reducing distractions and helping you prioritize healthier choices.

Measurement: Clear goals allow for effective tracking and measuring of progress, which in turn boosts confidence and accountability.

Long-term Success: Goals provide a roadmap for gradual and sustainable changes, ensuring that healthy eating becomes a lifestyle rather than a temporary fad.

Steps to Set Clear Goals for Healthy Eating Habits:

Define Your Purpose: Understand why you want to adopt healthier eating habits. Whether it's weight management, improved energy levels, or managing health conditions, a clear purpose will anchor your goals.

Be Specific: For instance, rather than saying "I want to eat healthier," specify, "I will consume at least five servings of vegetables daily for the next four weeks."

Start Small: Begin with manageable changes. Radical changes can be overwhelming and unsustainable. Gradual adjustments make it easier to adapt to new habits over time.

Focus on Nutrients: Instead of obsessing over calorie counts, focus on consuming nutrient-dense foods like fruits, vegetables, lean proteins, whole grains, and healthy fats

Stay Hydrated: Include adequate water intake as a part of your goals.

Minimize Processed Foods: Aim to minimize the consumption of processed and sugary foods.

Incorporate Variety: Include a variety of foods to ensure you receive a broad spectrum of nutrients. Experiment with different fruits, vegetables, grains, and proteins.

Allow Occasional Treats: It's important to enjoy treats occasionally to prevent feelings of deprivation. Moderation **is key to long-term success.**

Keep a Journal: Maintain a food journal to track what you eat, your mood, and any triggers for unhealthy eating. This can help you identify patterns and make necessary adjustments.

Seek Professional Guidance: If you have specific health goals or dietary restrictions, consider consulting a registered dietitian or nutritionist for personalized guidance.

Celebrate Milestones: Celebrate your achievements, no matter how small. This positive reinforcement can boost your motivation to continue on your healthy eating journey.

Remember, setting clear goals for healthy eating habits is a journey, not a destination. Be patient with yourself and open to making adjustments as needed. Regularly assess your progress, recalibrate your goals, and celebrate your successes along the way

Plan meals

Planning meals for healthy eating habits or a balanced diet is essential for maintaining overall well-being. A well-structured meal plan can help you achieve and sustain your health goals. Here's a comprehensive guide to help you create a plan that promotes healthy eating habits:

Set Clear Goals: Determine your health objectives, such as weight management, muscle gain, improved energy levels, or managing specific health conditions. Your goals will influence the composition of your meals.

Balanced Macronutrients: Focus on incorporating the three main macronutrients into your meals: carbohydrates, proteins, and fats. Opt for whole, unprocessed sources of each to ensure a balanced intake.

Include a Variety of Foods: Aim to consume a wide range of foods from all food groups: fruits, vegetables, lean proteins, whole grains, and healthy fats. This provides your body with essential nutrients.

Fruits and Vegetables: Make half your plate filled with colorful fruits and vegetables.

Lean Proteins: Incorporate lean sources of protein such as chicken, turkey, fish, beans, lentils, tofu, and low-fat dairy products. Protein are responsible for growing.

Eat Balance diet

Maintaining a balanced diet is essential for promoting a healthy eating habit and overall well-being. A balanced diet provides the body with the right combination of nutrients, including carbohydrates, proteins, fats, vitamins, and minerals, in appropriate proportions. Here's a comprehensive overview of the importance and components of a balanced diet:

1. Macronutrients:

Carbohydrate : They are responsible for production of energy for the body they include. Whole grains, fruits, vegetables, and legumes provide complex carbohydrates that release energy gradually, helping to regulate blood sugar levels.

Proteins: Proteins are crucial for tissue repair, immune function, and building enzymes and hormones. Sources of proteins include fish, milk, meat and egg

Fats: Healthy fats are essential for brain health, hormone production, and maintaining cell structure. Focus on unsaturated fats from sources like avocados, nuts, seeds, olive oil, and fatty fish. Limit saturated and trans fats found in fried and processed foods.

2. Micronutrients:

Vitamins: These are essential for various bodily functions, such as immune support, bone health, and energy production. Include a variety of fruits and vegetables to ensure a diverse intake of vitamins like A, C, D, E, and K.

Minerals: Minerals like calcium, magnesium, potassium, and iron are vital for bone health, nerve function, and blood production. Consume dairy products, leafy greens, nuts, seeds, and lean meats to ensure an adequate mineral intake.

3. Fiber:

Dietary fiber aids in digestion, prevents constipation, and supports gut health.sources of fibres include whole grains ,legumes and nuts

4. Hydration:

Water is essential for nearly every bodily function, from digestion and circulation to temperature regulation. Aim to drink an adequate amount of water throughout the day to stay properly hydration

6. Diversity:

Consuming a wide variety of foods ensures that you receive a spectrum of nutrients. Different foods offer different vitamins, minerals, and antioxidants, contributing to overall health.

7. Moderation:

While it's important to include a variety of foods, moderation is key. Even nutritious foods can become unhealthy when consumed excessively.

8. Avoid Excess Sugar, Salt, and Processed Foods:

Minimize the consumption of sugary drinks, snacks, and foods high in added sugars. Similarly, limit sodium intake by reducing processed and fast foods.

9. Personalization:

Everyone's nutritional needs are unique. Consider factors such as age, gender, activity level, and any specific health conditions when planning your balanced diet.

10. Consistency:

Developing healthy eating habits requires consistency over time. Aim to make balanced eating a lifelong practice rather than a short-term fix.

In conclusion, a balanced diet is the foundation of a healthy eating habit. It provides the body with the necessary nutrients to function optimally, supports overall well-being, and reduces the risk of chronic diseases. By including a variety of nutrient-rich foods in appropriate proportions, staying hydrated, and practicing moderation, you can cultivate a sustainable and health-promoting eating routine.

Choose Whole Food

Choosing whole foods is an essential aspect of maintaining a healthy and balanced diet. Whole foods are foods that are as close to their natural state as possible, and they have not been processed or refined extensively. These foods retain their natural nutrients, fiber, and health-promoting compounds, making them an integral part of a nutritious diet. Here are some key reasons and guidelines for choosing whole foods:

Benefits of Choosing Whole Foods:

35

Nutrient Density: Whole foods are rich in essential nutrients such as vitamins, minerals, and antioxidants. These nutrients are vital for various bodily functions, including metabolism, immune system support, and overall well-being.

Fiber Content: Whole foods, such as whole grains, fruits, vegetables, and legumes, are high in dietary fiber.

Natural Energy: Whole foods provide a steady source of energy due to their balanced composition of macronutrients. They are less likely to cause rapid spikes and crashes in blood sugar levels compared to processed foods.

Gut Health: Many whole foods contain prebiotics and probiotics that support a healthy gut microbiome. A diverse and well-balanced gut microbiome is linked to improved digestion, immunity, and mental health.

Reduced Added Sugars and Sodium: Whole foods typically have lower levels of added sugars and sodium compared to processed foods, which is beneficial for heart health and preventing chronic diseases.

Guidelines for Choosing Whole Foods:

Whole Grains: Choose whole grains like brown rice, quinoa, whole wheat, oats, and barley instead of refined grains like white rice or white bread. Whole grains retain their bran and germ, which are rich in nutrients and fiber.

Lean Proteins: Opt for lean sources of protein such as lean meats, poultry, fish, eggs, tofu, legumes, and nuts.

Minimally Processed Foods: Select foods with minimal processing. For example, plain yogurt instead of flavored yogurt with added sugars, and whole fruits instead of fruit juices.

Read Labels: When choosing packaged foods, read ingredient lists and nutrition labels. Look for shorter ingredient lists with recognizable whole-food ingredients. Be cautious of added sugars, artificial additives, and high levels of sodium.

Cook at Home:

Preparing food at home gives you the ability to have measure the ingredients and cooking procedures It's a great way to incorporate more whole foods into your diet.

Limit Highly Processed Foods:

Highly processed foods often contain unhealthy trans fats, excessive sugars, and sodium. Limit or avoid items like sugary snacks, sugary beverages, and heavily processed convenience foods.

Hydration:

Drink plenty of water and limit sugary drinks. Water is the best choice for staying hydrated without added sugars or artificial ingredients.

Variety:

Aim for a diverse diet that includes a variety of whole foods. Different foods offer different nutrients, ensuring you receive a balanced intake of essential vitamins and minerals.

Incorporating a wide range of whole foods into your diet can help you achieve and maintain good health. By making mindful choices and focusing on natural, unprocessed options, you can provide your body with the essential nutrients it needs to thrive.

Food, Groups, and Function

Food is not just sustenance; it is a rich tapestry of flavors, textures, and nutrients that fuel our bodies and nourish our souls. Our diets are composed of various food groups, each with its own nature, function, and unique characteristics. In this exploration of food groups, we'll delve into the intricate world of nutrition and discover the vital roles these groups play in maintaining our health.

1. Fruits

Nature: Fruits are the sweet and colorful gems of nature. They encompass a vast variety, from apples to zucchinis, each offering distinct flavors and nutritional profiles.

Function: Fruits are nature's dessert, brimming with vitamins, minerals, fiber, and antioxidants. They help boost our immune system, support digestion, and keep our skin radiant. Their natural sugars provide a quick energy source.

Unique Characteristics: Some fruits, like berries, are packed with antioxidants, protecting our cells from damage. Citrus fruits, such as oranges and lemons, are rich in vitamin C, vital for collagen production and immune health.

2. Vegetables

Nature: Vegetables are the green powerhouses of our plates. They come in various forms, including leafy greens, root vegetables, and cruciferous veggies like broccoli and cauliflower.

Function: Vegetables are a treasure trove of essential nutrients. They provide vitamins, minerals, fiber, and phytonutrients that support various bodily functions. Leafy greens are rich in iron and calcium, while carrots offer a hefty dose of vitamin A for healthy vision.

Unique Characteristics: Cruciferous vegetables, such as kale and Brussels sprouts, contain compounds that help detoxify the body. Spinach and Swiss chard are excellent sources of folate, essential for cell division and growth.

3. Grains

Nature: Grains are the starchy, hearty foundation of many diets worldwide. They encompass cereals like wheat, rice, oats, and pseudo cereals like quinoa.

Function: Grains are a primary source of carbohydrates, providing energy for our bodies. They also offer fiber, B vitamins, and essential minerals. Whole grains, like brown rice and whole wheat bread, are rich in fiber, aiding digestion and promoting fullness.

Unique Characteristics: Quinoa, classified as a pseudo cereal, is gluten-free and contains all nine essential amino acids, making it a complete protein source. Oats contain beta-glucans, which help lower cholesterol levels.

4. Protein Foods

Nature: Protein foods encompass both animal and plant-based sources. Animal sources include meat, poultry, fish, and dairy products, while plant-based options consist of beans, lentils, tofu, and nuts.

Function: Proteins are the building blocks of life. They are essential for tissue repair, immune function, and the production of enzymes and hormones. Animal-based proteins are complete proteins, containing all essential amino acids, while plant-based proteins often need to be combined to achieve this completeness.

Unique Characteristics: Salmon, a fatty fish, provides omega-3 fatty acids, beneficial for heart and brain health. Legumes like chickpeas are rich in plant-based protein and fiber, promoting satiety and digestive health.

5. Dairy and Dairy Alternatives

Nature: Dairy products originate from milk, typically from cows, but can also come from goats and sheep. Dairy alternatives, like almond and soy milk, are plant-based alternatives designed to mimic the taste and texture of dairy.

Function: Dairy is a powerhouse of calcium, crucial for strong bones and teeth. Dairy alternatives are often fortified with calcium and vitamin D.

Unique Characteristics: Greek yogurt is a dairy product known for its high protein content and probiotics that support gut health. Almond milk is low in calories and suitable for those with lactose intolerance.

6. Fats and Oils

Nature: Fats and oils are a diverse group, including butter, olive oil, avocado, and fatty fish like salmon.

Function: Fats serve as a concentrated source of energy and are essential for the absorption of fat-soluble vitamins (A, D, E, and K). Unsaturated fats, like those found in olive oil and avocados, support heart health.

Unique Characteristics: Extra virgin olive oil is rich in monounsaturated fats and antioxidants, which have been linked to lower rates of heart disease. Fatty fish, like salmon and mackerel, contain omega-3 fatty acids that reduce inflammation and support brain health.

7. Sweets and Treats

Nature: Sweets and treats are the indulgent side of our diets, encompassing chocolates, candies, cakes, and other sugary delights.

Function: While these foods aren't considered essential for our diets, they certainly provide enjoyment and satisfaction. In moderation, they can be a source of comfort and celebration.

Unique Characteristics: Dark chocolate contains antioxidants called flavonoids, which may have heart-protective benefits when consumed in moderation. Some desserts, like fruit salads, offer sweetness alongside the benefits of fruits.

In conclusion, the world of food groups is a symphony of flavors and nutrients. Each group plays a unique role in our nutrition, offering a range of essential components that keep our bodies functioning optimally. Understanding the nature and function of these groups empowers us to make informed choices, creating a harmonious relationship between our plates and our well-being

Chapter 3

Mindful Eating

Mindful eating is a practice that encourages individuals to pay full attention to their eating experiences, fostering a deeper connection between their mind and body during meals. The aim of mindful eating is to cultivate a healthier relationship with food, promote better digestion, and ultimately support a balanced and nutritious diet. Here's a comprehensive overview of mindful eating and its benefits for developing healthy eating habits:

1. Present Moment Awareness:

Mindful eating involves being fully present in the moment while eating. This means paying attention to the sensory experiences of eating, such as the taste, smell, texture, and appearance of the food. By focusing on the present moment, individuals can avoid distractions, like electronic devices or stressful thoughts, that can lead to overeating or poor food choices.

2. Savoring the Experience:

Mindful eating encourages individuals to savor each bite of food, enjoying the flavors and textures. By doing so, they can derive greater satisfaction from smaller portions and develop an enhanced appreciation for the food they consume.

3. Eating with Intention:

Mindful eating encourages individuals to eat with intention and purpose. Before eating, one should assess their hunger levels and make conscious choices about what and how much to eat, based on their body's needs.

4. Listening to Hunger and Fullness Cues:

Mindful eating involves tuning into the body's hunger and fullness cues. This prevents overeating and encourages individuals to stop eating when they feel comfortably satisfied, rather than eating until they are overly full.

5. Emotional Awareness:

Mindful eating also addresses emotional eating by helping individuals recognize their emotions and understand whether they're eating in response to genuine hunger or other feelings, such as stress, boredom, or sadness.

6. Non-Judgmental Attitude:

Mindful eating promotes self-compassion and a non-judgmental attitude towards food choices. Instead of labeling foods as "good" or "bad," individuals learn to view them as nourishment and make choices based on what their body needs.

7. Improved Digestion:

Being mindful while eating can positively impact digestion. Chewing food thoroughly and eating slowly aids in the breakdown of food, making it easier for the body to absorb nutrients.

8. Portion Control:

Mindful eating naturally encourages portion control, as individuals become more attuned to their body's cues and eat only until they are satisfied.

9. Weight Management:

Developing mindful eating habits can support weight management by reducing overeating and promoting a balanced approach to eating. This approach minimizes the likelihood of restrictive diets, which can lead to unhealthy eating patterns.

10. Enhanced Well-Being:

Mindful eating is linked to improved overall well-being. It can reduce stress related to food choices, foster a positive body image, and contribute to a healthier relationship with food.

11. Mind-Body Connection:

By engaging in mindful eating, individuals establish a stronger connection between their mind and body. This heightened awareness can extend beyond meal times and influence other aspects of their lives.

12. Gradual Change:

Developing mindful eating habits takes time and practice. It's about making small, sustainable changes to eating behaviors rather than drastic, short-term shifts.

Incorporating mindful eating into daily routines can lead to a more balanced and healthy approach to eating. By paying attention to the present moment, understanding hunger cues, and making intentional choices, individuals can foster a positive relationship with food and achieve long-term well-being.

Fiber Intake

carbohydrate found in plant-based foods that the body cannot fully digest. It offers a wide array of health benefits that contribute to overall well-being. Here's a comprehensive look at how fiber intake supports a healthy eating habit:

Digestive Health: Fiber plays a pivotal role in maintaining optimal digestive health. Insoluble fiber, found in foods like whole grains, nuts, and vegetables, helps prevent gastrointestinal issues by ensuring that food moves efficiently through the digestive tract.

Weight Management: Including fiber-rich foods in your diet can aid in weight management. High-fiber foods are often less calorie-dense and more filling, helping you feel satisfied with smaller portions. Fiber also slows down the digestion process, extending the feeling of fullness and reducing the likelihood of overeating.

Blood Sugar Regulation: Soluble fiber, found in foods like oats, beans, and fruits, can help regulate blood sugar levels by slowing down the absorption of sugar.

Heart Health: Fiber intake is associated with a lower risk of heart disease. Soluble fiber helps lower levels of LDL cholesterol (often referred to as "bad" cholesterol) by binding to cholesterol particles and removing them from the body. A diet rich in fiber can also help reduce blood pressure and inflammation, further supporting cardiovascular health.

Gut Microbiota: Fiber acts as a prebiotic, providing nourishment to beneficial gut bacteria. A healthy gut microbiome is linked to various aspects of health, including immunity, mood regulation, and even weight management.

Colon Health: A diet high in fiber has been linked to a reduced risk of developing colorectal cancer. Fiber helps maintain a healthy colon environment by promoting regular bowel movements and minimizing exposure to harmful substances.

Satiation and Appetite Control: Fiber-rich foods take longer to chew and digest, providing a sense of fullness and satisfaction. This can help prevent excessive snacking between meals and contribute to better appetite control.

Nutrient Absorption: Fiber can enhance the absorption of certain nutrients, such as calcium and magnesium, by promoting a healthier intestinal environment. This ensures that the body can effectively utilize the nutrients present in the foods you consume.

Lowering Inflammation: Chronic inflammation is associated with various health issues, including heart disease and certain autoimmune conditions. A diet high in fiber-rich foods, such as fruits, vegetables, and whole grains, can help reduce inflammation and support overall immune function.

Balanced Blood Lipids: Fiber aids in maintaining balanced levels of triglycerides and other blood lipids, contributing to a healthier lipid profile.

To incorporate more fiber into your diet, focus on consuming whole, minimally processed foods. Include a variety of fruits, vegetables, legumes, whole grains, nuts, and seeds. Gradually increase your fiber intake to allow your digestive system to adjust. Remember to drink plenty of water, as fiber absorbs water and can lead to bloating or discomfort if not consumed with adequate fluids.

In conclusion, fiber intake is a cornerstone of a healthy eating habit. Its benefits extend beyond digestive health to encompass weight management, heart health, blood sugar regulation, and more. By prioritizing fiber-rich foods, you can significantly enhance your overall well-being and reduce the risk of various chronic diseases.

Incorporating an adequate amount of dietary fiber into your eating habits is essential for maintaining a healthy lifestyle. Fiber is a type of carbohydrate found in plant-based foods that the body cannot fully digest. It offers a wide array of health benefits that contribute to overall well-being. Here's a comprehensive look at how fiber intake supports a healthy eating habit:

Digestive Health: Fiber plays a pivotal role in maintaining optimal digestive health. It adds bulk to the stool, preventing constipation and promoting regular bowel movements. Insoluble fiber, found in foods like whole grains, nuts, and vegetables, helps prevent gastrointestinal issues by ensuring that food moves efficiently through the digestive tract.

Weight Management: Including fiber-rich foods in your diet can aid in weight management. High-fiber foods are often less calorie-dense and more filling, helping you feel satisfied with smaller portions. Fiber also slows down the digestion process, extending the feeling of fullness and reducing the likelihood of overeating.

Blood Sugar Regulation: Soluble fiber, found in foods like oats, beans, and fruits, can help regulate blood sugar levels by slowing down the absorption of sugar.

Heart Health: Fiber intake is associated with a lower risk of heart disease. Soluble fiber helps lower levels of LDL cholesterol (often referred to as "bad" cholesterol) by binding to cholesterol particles and removing them from the body.

Gut Microbiota: Fiber acts as a prebiotic, providing nourishment to beneficial gut bacteria. A healthy gut microbiome is linked to various aspects of health, including immunity, mood regulation, and even weight management.

Colon Health: A diet high in fiber has been linked to a reduced risk of developing colorectal cancer. Fiber helps maintain a healthy colon environment by promoting regular bowel movements and minimizing exposure to harmful substances.

Satiation and Appetite Control: Fiber-rich foods take longer to chew and digest, providing a sense of fullness and satisfaction.

Nutrient Absorption: Fiber can enhance the absorption of certain nutrients, such as calcium and magnesium, by promoting a healthier intestinal environment. This ensures that the body can effectively utilize the nutrients present in the foods you consume.

Lowering Inflammation: Chronic inflammation is associated with various health issues, including heart disease and certain autoimmune conditions. A diet high in fiber-rich foods, such as fruits, vegetables, and whole grains, can help reduce inflammation and support overall immune function.

In conclusion, fiber intake is a cornerstone of a healthy eating habit. Its benefits extend beyond digestive health to encompass weight management, heart health, blood sugar regulation, and more. By prioritizing fiber-rich foods, you can significantly enhance your overall well-being and reduce the risk of various chronic diseases

Limit Sugar

Sugars are not normally found in foods. These sugars contribute to the sweetness, flavor, and texture of many processed foods and beverages, but their excessive consumption can have detrimental effects on health.

Health Concerns:

Weight Gain and Obesity: Added sugars provide extra calories without significant nutritional value, leading to an increase in overall calorie intake. This can contribute to weight gain and obesity, as excess calories are stored as fat.

Type 2 Diabetes: High intake of added sugars can lead to insulin resistance, a condition where cells become less responsive to the effects of insulin.

Cardiovascular Health: Excessive sugar intake has been linked to an increased risk of heart disease. Diets high in added sugars can raise triglyceride levels, blood pressure, and contribute to inflammation.

Metabolic Syndrome: A combination of conditions, including high blood pressure, high blood sugar, excess abdominal fat, and abnormal cholesterol levels, can be exacerbated by excessive sugar consumption.

Healthy Fats

Healthy fats, also known as unsaturated fats, are essential components of a balanced diet that contribute to overall well-being. Unlike saturated and trans fats, which are associated with negative health effects, healthy fats offer a range of benefits for the body.

There are two main types of healthy fats: monounsaturated fats and polyunsaturated fats. Monounsaturated fats are found in foods like olive oil, avocados, nuts (such as almonds, cashews, and peanuts), and seeds. They have been linked to improved heart health by helping to lower bad cholesterol levels (LDL cholesterol) while maintaining or even increasing good cholesterol levels (HDL cholesterol). Additionally, monounsaturated fats provide a source of energy, aid in nutrient absorption, and support cell growth.

Polyunsaturated fats are divided into two categories: omega-3 fatty acids and omega-6 fatty acids. Omega-3s are abundant in fatty fish (such as salmon, mackerel, and sardines), flaxseeds, chia seeds, and walnuts. They are renowned for their anti-inflammatory properties, which play a crucial role in reducing the risk of chronic diseases like heart disease, arthritis, and even some types of cancer. Omega-3s also support brain health, cognitive function, and mood regulation.

Omega-6 fatty acids are found in vegetable oils (such as soybean, corn, and sunflower oils) and nuts. They are important for maintaining healthy skin, hair, and bone health, as well as supporting the overall functioning of cells in the body. However, it's essential to strike a balance between omega-3 and omega-6 consumption, as excessive omega-6 intake relative to omega-3s could potentially contribute to inflammation.

Incorporating healthy fats into your diet is relatively easy. Substituting saturated fats (found in animal products and some processed foods) with sources of healthy fats can lead to improved heart health and reduced risk of chronic diseases. Cooking with olive oil, snacking on nuts or seeds, enjoying fatty fish, and using avocados in salads are all simple ways to include these fats in your meals.

It's important to note that while healthy fats offer numerous benefits, they are calorie-dense. As with any nutrient, moderation is key. Aim to replace unhealthy fats in your diet with healthier options, rather than simply adding more fats to your intake. Balancing your overall diet, exercising regularly, and consulting with a healthcare professional or registered dietitian can help you make informed choices that support your health and well-being.

Protein Source

Protein are essential components of a balanced diet, playing a crucial role in maintaining various bodily functions and promoting overall health. Proteins are made up of amino acids, which are the building blocks that the body uses to repair tissues, produce enzymes and hormones, support the immune system, and facilitate various physiological processes.

Protein sources can be classified into two main categories: animal-based and plant-based.

Animal-Based Protein Sources:

Seafood: Fish and seafood are low in fat and high in protein, making them excellent choices for obtaining essential omega-3 fatty acids.

Dairy Products: Milk, cheese, yogurt, and eggs are rich in protein and often contain other important nutrients like calcium and vitamin D.

Plant-Based Protein Sources:

Plant-based proteins may lack some of the essential amino acids individually, but they can be combined strategically to create complete protein profiles. Some common plant-based protein sources include:

Legumes: Beans (black beans, kidney beans, chickpeas, etc.), lentils, and peas are excellent sources of protein, fiber, and various vitamins and minerals.

Nuts and Seeds: Almonds, peanuts, chia seeds, flaxseeds, and sunflower seeds provide protein, healthy fats, and other nutrients.

Whole Grains: Quinoa, brown rice, oats, and whole wheat products offer protein along with complex carbohydrates and fiber.

Soy Products: Tofu, tempeh, and edamame are derived from soybeans and provide a complete protein profile. They are also rich in phytonutrients.

It's important to note that while animal-based proteins can be high in saturated fats, which can contribute to heart disease, plant-based proteins tend to be lower in saturated fats and can offer additional health benefits due to their fiber and antioxidant content. However, they might lack certain nutrients like vitamin B12 and omega-3 fatty acids, which are more abundant in animal-based sources.

A well-balanced diet often includes a mix of both animal-based and plant-based protein sources, tailored to individual dietary preferences and health goals. Whether you choose to get your protein from animal or plant sources, focusing on variety and moderation is key to obtaining a wide range of essential

Cultivating a Healthy Eating Habit

<u>*Chapter 4*</u>

Eating Colorful Vegetable

Eating a diet rich in vegetables and fruits is essential for maintaining good health. These nutrient-dense foods are packed with vitamins, minerals, antioxidants, and dietary fiber, which contribute to overall well-being and help reduce the risk of chronic diseases. Here's a comprehensive look at eating healthy vegetables and fruits, including meal frequency:

Benefits of Eating Vegetables and Fruits

Nutrient Content:

Vegetables and fruits are low in calories and high in essential nutrients like vitamins A, C, and K, as well as minerals like potassium and magnesium. These nutrients support various bodily functions, including immune function, bone health, and heart health.

Antioxidants: Many fruits and vegetables are rich in antioxidants, which help combat oxidative stress and protect cells from damage caused by free radicals.

Fiber: Both vegetables and fruits are excellent sources of dietary fiber, which aids digestion, promotes a feeling of fullness, and helps regulate blood sugar levels. Fiber also supports a healthy gut microbiome.

Hydration: Fruits and vegetables have a high water content, contributing to hydration and overall fluid balance in the body.

Weight Management: Incorporating plenty of vegetables and fruits into your diet can help with weight management, as they are low in calories and high in fiber, promoting a feeling of satiety.

Meal Frequency:

When it comes to meal frequency, there isn't a one-size-fits-all answer, as individual needs and preferences vary.

Daily Intake: Aim to consume a variety of vegetables and fruits every day to ensure you're getting a wide range of nutrients. The USDA recommends filling half your plate with fruits and vegetables at each meal.

Cultivating a Healthy Eating Habit

Portion Sizes: Include at least 5 servings of vegetables and fruits per day. A serving is generally considered to be one cup of leafy greens or half a cup of chopped vegetables or fruits.

Snacking: Incorporate vegetables and fruits into your snacks. Snacking on fresh fruits, carrot sticks, celery, or bell pepper slices can be a healthier alternative to processed snacks.

Meal Balance: Integrate vegetables and fruits into every meal to create a well-rounded diet. Add berries to your breakfast, include a variety of veggies in your lunch and dinner, and have fruits as dessert or snacks.

Colorful Variety: Aim to eat a variety of colorful fruits and vegetables.

Frozen and Canned Options: If fresh produce is not readily available, frozen and canned options can still offer nutritional benefits. Just be mindful of added sugars or sodium in canned versions.

Cooking Methods: Experiment with different cooking methods, such as steaming, roasting, sautéing, and grilling, to make vegetables more enjoyable.

Diverse Choices: Choose a diverse range of vegetables and fruits to ensure you're getting a broad spectrum of nutrients. Include leafy greens, cruciferous vegetables, berries, citrus fruits, and more.

Incorporating vegetables and fruits into your meals and snacks regularly can contribute significantly to your overall health. Remember that balance and variety are key, and it's important to enjoy the process of exploring different options to find what suits your taste and lifestyle best.

Frequent Meal

Meal frequency" refers to the number of times a person eats in a day. It's an aspect of dietary habits that can impact overall health and well-being. The concept of meal frequency has been a topic of interest and research in the field of nutrition for many years.

There's no one-size-fits-all answer when it comes to how often someone should eat in a day, as it can vary based on individual preferences, daily routine, cultural practices, and dietary goals. Here are a few points to consider about meal frequency:

Traditional Approach: The traditional three-meal-a-day approach (breakfast, lunch, and dinner) is common in many cultures. This pattern can provide structure to the day and may help regulate hunger levels.

Snacking: In recent years, snacking between meals has become more common. Snacks can provide energy boosts between meals and help prevent overeating during main meals. However, the quality of snacks matters; opting for nutrient-dense snacks is important.

Meal Timing: The timing of meals can affect factors like metabolism, blood sugar levels, and digestion. Some people prefer eating smaller meals more frequently throughout the day, while others find larger meals at specific times more satisfying.

Hunger and Satiety: Paying attention to your body's hunger and fullness cues is crucial. Eating when you're hungry and stopping when you're satisfied can help prevent overeating and promote a healthier relationship with food.

Athletes and Active Individuals: Athletes and those with high energy expenditure might benefit from consuming multiple meals or snacks to support their energy needs and recovery.

Weight Management: For weight management, some studies suggest that spreading caloric intake across multiple meals might help control hunger and prevent extreme fluctuations in blood sugar levels.

Intermittent Fasting: This eating pattern involves alternating between periods of eating and fasting. It has gained popularity for potential health benefits, although individual responses vary.

Digestion and Nutrient Absorption: Some people find that **eating** smaller, more frequent meals helps with digestion, while others prefer larger meals that give their digestive system more time to rest between meals.

Health Conditions: People with certain health conditions, such as diabetes, might need to consider meal frequency and timing to manage blood sugar levels.

Mindful Eating: Regardless of meal frequency, practicing mindful eating—paying attention to the flavors, textures, and enjoyment of food—can foster a healthier relationship with meals.

In conclusion, meal frequency is a flexible aspect of nutrition that can be tailored to an individual's preferences, lifestyle, and health goals. There's no one "right" way to approach it, but listening to your body's cues, choosing nutrient-dense foods, and maintaining a balanced diet are key factors for overall well-being. It's always a good idea to consult with a registered dietitian or healthcare professional to determine the best meal frequency strategy for your specific needs.

Reading label

Reading labels is a crucial skill when it comes to maintaining a healthy eating habit. Labels provide valuable information about the nutritional content of the food you're consuming, helping you make informed choices that align with your health goals. Here's a comprehensive guide on how to read labels for a healthy eating habit

Calories: The calorie count per serving tells you how much energy you'll gain from consuming that portion. Keep in mind your daily caloric needs and balance your intake accordingly.

Macronutrients:

Fat: Check the total fat content and the type of fats present (saturated, trans, unsaturated). Aim to limit saturated and trans fats, while focusing on healthier unsaturated fats.

Carbohydrates: Look at the total carbohydrates, including dietary fiber and sugars. Favor foods higher in dietary fiber and lower in added sugars.

Protein: Monitor the protein content, which is essential for muscle repair and overall body function.

Dietary Fiber: Adequate fiber intake aids digestion, promotes satiety, and can help manage weight.

Added Sugars: Differentiate between natural sugars (found in fruits) and added sugars. Limit foods with high amounts of added sugars, as excessive consumption is linked to various health issues.

Sodium (Salt): Excessive sodium intake can lead to high blood pressure. Be cautious of products with high sodium content, especially if you have a history of hypertension.

Vitamins and Minerals: Labels often list the percentage of daily value (%DV) for certain vitamins and minerals. These can help you assess whether a product contributes to your daily nutrient needs.

Allergens: Labels typically highlight common allergens such as nuts, dairy, soy, and wheat. If you have allergies or sensitivities, ensure the product is safe for you.

Health Claims: Be cautious of marketing terms like "low-fat," "reduced-sugar," or "natural." These claims may not always reflect the product's overall healthfulness. Always verify by checking the actual nutritional values.

Comparing Similar Products: When choosing between similar products, compare their labels. Opt for options with better nutritional profiles, like lower saturated fat, sugar, and sodium content.

Consider Your Goals: Tailor your label reading to your health goals. If you're aiming for weight loss, focus on portion size and calorie content. If you're looking to increase muscle mass, prioritize protein content.

Remember that while reading labels is a valuable tool, it's also important to maintain a balanced diet filled with whole, unprocessed foods. Labels provide information, but your overall dietary choices play a significant role in achieving and maintaining a healthy eating habit.

Cook at home

Cooking at home offers several benefits for developing good nutrition habits. Here's a comprehensive look at how cooking at home can contribute to a healthier lifestyle:

Power over your ingredients :

This allows you to choose fresh, whole foods and avoid additives, preservatives, and excessive amounts of salt, sugar, and unhealthy fats that are often found in processed and restaurant foods.

Balanced Meals: Preparing meals at home enables you to create balanced dishes that include a variety of nutrients. You can include a mix of lean proteins, whole grains, vegetables, and fruits to ensure that your meals are nutritionally well-rounded.

Portion Control: Home-cooked meals allow you to control portion sizes, which is crucial for managing calorie intake.

Customization: Cooking at home lets you tailor meals to meet your specific dietary needs and preferences.

Whether you're following a specific diet (e.g., vegetarian, gluten-free) or catering to allergies, you can ensure that your meals align with your nutritional requirements.

Less Hidden Calories: Restaurant and packaged foods often contain hidden calories from added fats, sugars, and portion sizes that are larger than what you might consume at home. Cooking your own meals allows you to keep track of calorie content more accurately.

Higher Nutrient Retention: The longer food is exposed to heat and light, the more nutrients it can lose. Cooking at home usually involves shorter cooking times and more careful handling of ingredients, helping to retain more of their original nutrients.

Learning About Nutrition: Cooking at home encourages you to learn about different foods and their nutritional profiles. This knowledge empowers you to make informed choices about what you eat and to create meals that fulfill your body's nutritional needs.

Mindful Eating: Preparing your own meals promotes mindfulness around eating. You're more likely to savor your food and pay attention to hunger and fullness cues, leading to healthier eating habits.

Family Engagement: Cooking at home can involve family members, creating an opportunity to bond and teach valuable cooking and nutrition skills to children. When kids are involved in meal preparation, they're more likely to develop healthy eating habits themselves.

Cost Savings: Preparing meals at home can be more cost-effective than dining out. This allows you to invest in high-quality ingredients, including fresh produce and lean proteins, which contribute to a balanced diet.

Experimentation: Cooking at home encourages culinary experimentation. You can try new recipes, cooking techniques, and ingredients, which can expand your palate and encourage you to incorporate a wider range of nutrient-rich foods into your diet.

Reduced Dependence on Processed Foods: Processed foods often lack essential nutrients and can contribute to health issues over time. Cooking at home reduces your reliance on these items, promoting a diet rich in whole, natural foods.

In conclusion, cooking at home plays a vital role in developing good nutrition habits by allowing you to control ingredients, portion sizes, and meal balance. It fosters a deeper understanding of nutrition, promotes mindful eating, and offers opportunities for creativity in the kitchen. By making cooking a regular part of your routine, you can enjoy the numerous health benefits associated with a well-rounded and nutritious diet.

Chapter 5

Limiting Processed Food

Limiting processed meals can greatly contribute to promoting a healthy diet. Processed meals, often high in added sugars, unhealthy fats, and sodium, can have detrimental effects on overall health. Here's a comprehensive overview of how reducing the consumption of processed meals can positively impact one's **diet:**

Nutrient Density: Whole, unprocessed foods like fruits, vegetables, whole grains, lean proteins, and nuts are rich in essential nutrients such as vitamins, minerals, fiber, and antioxidants. By consuming more of these foods and fewer processed meals, individuals can ensure they're getting a broader range of nutrients necessary for optimal health.

Reduced Added Sugars: Many processed meals contain hidden sugars, which can contribute to weight gain, insulin resistance, and other metabolic issues. By choosing whole foods, individuals can control their sugar intake and reduce the risk of developing conditions like type 2 diabetes.

Healthy Fats: Processed meals often contain unhealthy trans fats and excessive saturated fats. Opting for whole foods allows individuals to consume healthier fats, such as those found in avocados, nuts, seeds, and fatty fish, which can support heart health and overall well-being.

Lower Sodium Intake: Processed meals tend to be high in sodium, which can lead to hypertension and other cardiovascular problems. Preparing meals from scratch allows individuals to regulate their salt intake and make healthier choices for flavoring, like herbs and spices.

Fiber Content: Whole foods are generally higher in dietary fiber, which supports digestive health, helps control blood sugar levels, and promotes a feeling of fullness. Processed meals often lack sufficient fiber, contributing to overeating and digestive issues.

Control over Ingredients: Preparing meals at home provides control over ingredient quality and allows for customization based on personal dietary needs and preferences. This can be especially beneficial for individuals with allergies, intolerances, or specific nutritional goals.

Mindful Eating: Preparing meals from whole foods encourages mindfulness about food choices. This practice can help individuals become more attuned to their hunger and fullness cues, leading to better portion control and a healthier relationship with food.

Weight Management: Processed meals are often energy-dense and lack nutritional value, which can contribute to overconsumption of calories. Choosing whole, nutrient-dense foods can help manage weight by providing essential nutrients without excessive calories.

Long-Term Health Benefits: A diet rich in whole foods has been associated with a lower risk of chronic diseases such as heart disease, obesity, and certain types of cancer. Avoiding processed meals is a proactive step toward better long-term health.

Improved Energy Levels: The balanced nutrients found in whole foods can provide sustained energy throughout the day, whereas processed meals high in sugar and unhealthy fats can lead to energy crashes and fatigue.

Positive Impact on Mental Health: A well-balanced diet consisting of whole foods can positively affect mood and cognitive function. Nutrients like omega-3 fatty acids, B vitamins, and antioxidants support brain health and emotional well-being.

Culinary Skills: Preparing meals from scratch can foster an interest in cooking, leading to the development of valuable culinary skills and an appreciation for the art of cooking and creating nutritious meals.

In conclusion, limiting processed meals and prioritizing whole, unprocessed foods can have a significant impact on overall health and well-being. The nutrient density, reduced added sugars, healthy fats, lower sodium intake, and other benefits of consuming whole foods contribute to a healthier lifestyle, making it an essential practice for promoting optimal health.

Incorporate Variety

Incorporating variety into your eating habits is crucial for maintaining a balanced and healthy diet. Not only does it provide a wide range of nutrients, but it also keeps your meals interesting and enjoyable. Here's a comprehensive guide on how to incorporate variety to promote a good eating habit:

Choose a Colorful Plate: Include a variety of colorful fruits and vegetables in your meals. Different colors often indicate different nutrients, so aim to have a mix of greens, reds, yellows, and purples on your plate.

Explore Different Food Groups: Incorporate foods from all the major food groups: fruits, vegetables, whole grains, lean proteins, and healthy fats. This ensures you're getting a diverse array of nutrients.

Rotate Proteins: Switch up your protein sources. Include lean meats, poultry, fish, beans, lentils, tofu, and nuts. This not only provides various nutrients but also prevents boredom with your meals.

Try New Whole Grains: Experiment with different whole grains like quinoa, brown rice, farro, and bulgur. These grains offer unique textures and flavors while delivering essential fiber and nutrients.

Seasonal Eating: Embrace seasonal produce. Fruits and vegetables are often more flavorful and nutrient-rich when they are in season. This also supports local agriculture and reduces the carbon footprint of your food choices.

Culinary Techniques: Try various cooking methods to enhance flavors. Roasting, grilling, steaming, and sautéing can bring out different qualities in ingredients.

Global Cuisine: Explore cuisines from around the world. Different cultures use diverse combinations of ingredients and spices, which can open up a world of flavors and textures to your palate.

Weekly Meal Planning: Plan your meals for the week ahead. This allows you to incorporate a variety of foods and ensures that you're not relying on the same ingredients repeatedly.

Snack Wisely: Choose a range of nutritious snacks. Mix fruits, veggies, yogurt, nuts, and whole-grain crackers to keep your energy levels steady between meals

Rotate Breakfast Options: Instead of having the same breakfast every day, switch between options like oatmeal, yogurt parfaits, smoothies, whole-grain toast with avocado, and scrambled eggs.

Salad Creations: Create diverse salads using a variety of greens, toppings, and dressings. Incorporate nuts, seeds, fruits, cheeses, and lean proteins to keep salads exciting.

Healthy Swaps: Make healthier ingredient substitutions. For example, replace white pasta with whole wheat or zucchini noodles, or swap regular rice with cauliflower rice.

Keep Healthy Snacks Handy: Keep a variety of healthy snacks within easy reach to avoid reaching for less nutritious options when hunger strikes.

Hydration Variety: Choose different beverages to stay hydrated. Include water, herbal teas, infused waters, and naturally flavored sparkling water.

Moderation is Key: While variety is important, moderation is also crucial. Overloading your plate with too many different foods can lead to excessive calorie intake.

Gradual Changes: Introduce new foods gradually. If you're trying to expand your palate, start with small portions and gradually increase as you become more comfortable with the taste.

Remember, the goal of incorporating variety is not only to improve your nutrition but also to make eating an enjoyable experience. Listen to your body, embrace new flavors, and have fun experimenting with different foods and recipes

Practice Consistency

Consistency is a key factor in promoting a healthy nutrition regimen. By consistently making nutritious food choices and maintaining a balanced diet, individuals can experience numerous benefits for their overall health and well-being. Here's a comprehensive overview of how consistency can promote healthy nutrition:

Establishing Good Habits: Consistency helps in establishing good eating habits. When individuals consistently choose healthy foods, they are more likely to create a routine of making nutritious choices, which becomes a natural part of their daily life.

Steady Nutrient Intake: Consistently consuming a variety of nutrient-rich foods ensures a steady intake of essential vitamins, minerals, and macronutrients. This supports the body's various functions, such as energy production, immune system function, and overall growth.

Maintaining Stable Energy Levels: Regularly eating balanced meals and snacks helps maintain stable blood sugar levels throughout the day. This prevents energy crashes and reduces the likelihood of overeating or making poor food choices due to extreme hunger.

Weight Management: Consistency in food choices and portion control plays a crucial role in weight management. When individuals consistently make healthy choices, they are more likely to control their calorie intake, which can contribute to achieving and maintaining a healthy weight.

Digestive Health: A consistent intake of fiber-rich foods, such as fruits, vegetables, and whole grains, supports digestive health. Fiber promotes regular bowel movements, prevents constipation, and maintains a healthy gut microbiome.

Reduced Risk of Chronic Diseases: A consistent intake of nutrient-dense foods, along with minimizing processed and sugary options, can help reduce the risk of chronic diseases such as heart disease, diabetes, and certain types of cancer.

Positive Impact on Mental Health: Consistently nourishing the body with wholesome foods can have a positive impact on mental health. Nutrients like omega-3 fatty acids, B vitamins, and antioxidants found in various foods support brain health and cognitive function.

Long-Term Sustainability: Consistency fosters a sustainable approach to nutrition. Extreme diets or sporadic unhealthy eating patterns are difficult to maintain in the long run. Consistently choosing nutritious foods allows for a more sustainable and enjoyable relationship with food.

Enhanced Athletic Performance: Athletes and active individuals benefit from consistent nutrition because it provides the energy and nutrients needed for optimal performance, endurance, and recovery.

Education and Mindfulness: Consistency encourages individuals to educate themselves about nutrition and make mindful choices. Over time, they become more aware of the nutritional value of different foods and can make informed decisions.

Routine and Meal Planning: Consistency promotes the development of meal planning and preparation routines. Planning meals ahead of time helps individuals make healthier choices and prevents last-minute unhealthy options.

Social and Environmental Impact: Making consistent choices that align with healthy nutrition not only benefits the individual but also has a positive impact on the environment and can influence others around them to adopt healthier habits.

In conclusion, consistency is the foundation of a healthy nutrition plan. By consistently making nutritious choices, individuals can establish good habits, maintain stable energy levels, manage weight, reduce the risk of chronic diseases, and experience positive effects on mental health. It's important to remember that consistency doesn't mean perfection—occasional indulgences are fine as long as they are balanced within an overall healthy eating pattern.

Seek Professional Guidance

Seeking professional guidance can play a crucial role in establishing and maintaining healthy eating habits and a balanced diet. Here's a comprehensive overview of how professional guidance can promise these benefits:

Personalized Approach: A registered dietitian or nutritionist can assess your individual needs, goals, medical history, and dietary preferences to create a personalized eating plan. This tailored approach ensures that your nutritional requirements are met, and you receive the right balance of nutrients.

Accurate Information: With the abundance of nutrition-related information available online and in media, it's easy to get confused. Professionals can provide evidence-based information and dispel myths, offering accurate advice on portion sizes, food choices, and dietary patterns.

Health Conditions Management: If you have specific health conditions like diabetes, heart disease, allergies, or gastrointestinal issues, a professional can design a diet that manages and improves your condition. They consider medical factors, creating a diet plan that aligns with your treatment and health goals.

Prevention of Nutritional Deficiencies: Professionals can help prevent deficiencies by identifying potential gaps in your diet and recommending appropriate supplements or food sources. This is particularly important for vegetarians, vegans, and those with restricted diets.

Behavioral Changes: Changing eating habits involves behavioral adjustments. A professional can provide strategies and support to help you make sustainable changes over time.

Education and Empowerment: Professionals empower you with knowledge about nutrient-rich foods, food labels, and meal planning. This education equips you to make informed decisions when shopping, cooking, and dining out, ensuring a consistent commitment to healthy eating.

Long-Term Success: Crash diets and extreme restrictions are rarely sustainable. Professionals emphasize gradual, sustainable changes that can be maintained over the long term. This approach prevents the cycle of yo-yo dieting and weight gain.

Support and Accountability: Regular appointments with a professional provide accountability and motivation. Knowing that you have someone to report to can encourage you to stick to your dietary goals and resist temptations.

Meal Planning and Preparation: Professionals can help you with meal planning, creating balanced meals that meet your nutritional needs. This can save you time, reduce stress, and prevent last-minute unhealthy food choices.

Mindful Eating: Professionals often promote mindful eating, which involves being present during meals, savoring each bite, and paying attention to hunger and fullness cues. This approach fosters a healthier relationship with food and reduces overeating.

Weight Management: If weight management is a goal, professionals can guide you towards achieving a healthy weight through a combination of balanced nutrition, exercise, and behavioral changes.

Adapting to Lifestyle Changes: Changes in life circumstances, such as pregnancy, aging, or shifts in activity levels, require adjustments in dietary habits. Professionals can help you adapt your diet to meet these changing needs.

In summary, seeking professional guidance for healthy eating habits and a balanced diet offers personalized advice, accurate information, and support for managing health conditions. It empowers you with knowledge, behavioral strategies, and the tools needed for long-term success. By addressing individual needs and providing ongoing guidance, professionals play a critical role in helping individuals achieve and maintain their health and wellness goals.

Listening To Your Body

Listening to your body is a fundamental aspect of promoting a healthy eating habit. In a world filled with fad diets and conflicting nutritional advice, tuning into your body's signals can guide you towards making informed food choices that support your overall well-being. Here's how actively listening to your body can help cultivate a balanced and sustainable approach to eating.

1. Recognizing Hunger and Fullness: One of the key components of healthy eating is understanding your body's hunger and fullness cues. Paying attention to sensations like a growling stomach or a subtle feeling of fullness can help you eat when you're genuinely hungry and stop when you're satisfied.

2. Identifying Cravings: Cravings are often your body's way of communicating specific nutrient needs. Craving chocolate might indicate a need for magnesium, while a hankering for salty foods could mean your body requires more electrolytes. Listening to these signals can help you choose nutrient-dense foods that address your body's requirements.

3. Differentiating Between Emotional and Physical Hunger: Emotional eating can lead to consuming excess calories and unhealthy food choices. Learning to distinguish between emotional hunger (triggered by stress, boredom, or sadness) and physical hunger enables you to address underlying emotions without using food as a coping mechanism.

4. Customizing Nutritional Intake: No one diet fits all. Each person's nutritional needs vary based on factors such as age, activity level, and metabolism. By tuning into your body's responses to different foods, you can customize your diet to match your unique requirements and preferences.

5. Enhancing Digestive Comfort: Listening to your body can help you identify foods that agree with your digestive system. Pay attention to how you feel after meals. If certain foods lead to bloating, discomfort, or digestive distress, you can make choices that support your gut health.

6. Mindful Eating: Mindful eating is about savoring each bite, being fully present during meals, and enjoying the sensory experience of food. This practice encourages you to slow down, chew thoroughly, and appreciate the flavors and textures of what you're eating. By doing so, you're more likely to recognize when you're satisfied, preventing overeating.

7. Adjusting Portion Sizes: Your body's energy needs change based on factors like physical activity and stress levels. Listening to your body allows you to adjust portion sizes accordingly. On days when you're more active, you might naturally crave more food, whereas when you're less active, smaller portions might suffice.

8. Long-Term Sustainability: Strict diets often lead to feelings of deprivation, making them difficult to maintain. Listening to your body helps you create a sustainable eating plan that aligns with your preferences and lifestyle. This increases the likelihood of sticking to healthier eating habits in the long run.

9. Building a Positive Relationship with Food: Viewing food as nourishment rather than the enemy promotes a positive relationship with what you eat. By honoring your body's signals, you reduce guilt associated with indulgent treats and develop a healthier attitude towards food.

10. Intuitive Eating: Intuitive eating is a philosophy that encourages you to trust your body's wisdom when it comes to food choices. It's about breaking free from diet culture and external rules and instead focusing on internal cues. This approach can lead to improved self-esteem and reduced stress related to food.

In conclusion, listening to your body is an essential component of cultivating a healthy eating habit. By recognizing hunger and fullness, differentiating between emotional and physical hunger, and tuning into cravings and digestive responses, you can make informed food choices that support your overall well-being. Embracing mindful eating, adjusting portion sizes, and adopting intuitive eating principles can lead to a sustainable, balanced approach to nourishing your body. Ultimately, the more you listen to your body, the more you empower yourself to make choices that promote long-lasting

health and vitality.

Proper Hydration

Hydration plays a crucial role in promoting healthy eating habits and overall well-being. While often overlooked, the connection between hydration and dietary choices is significant, and understanding this relationship can lead to improved health outcomes. In this essay, we will delve into the various ways in which hydration supports healthy eating habits and explore the science behind this connection.

Hydration is the process of providing your body with an adequate amount of fluids, primarily water, to maintain its essential functions. It is well-established that water is vital for overall health, as it constitutes a substantial portion of our bodies and is involved in numerous physiological processes. The importance of hydration becomes even more apparent when considering its impact on eating behaviors.

Firstly, staying hydrated can help regulate appetite and prevent overeating. Our bodies often confuse thirst with hunger, leading to unnecessary consumption of calories when what we truly need is fluids. By maintaining proper hydration levels, individuals can accurately interpret their body's signals and differentiate between thirst and hunger. This awareness can help prevent mindless snacking and overeating, promoting a more mindful and balanced approach to eating.

Secondly, drinking water before meals can aid in portion control. Studies have shown that having a glass of water before a meal can create a sense of fullness, resulting in reduced food intake. This can be particularly beneficial for those trying to manage their weight or control their calorie intake. Moreover, water-rich foods like fruits and vegetables can also contribute to hydration while providing essential nutrients, further supporting a healthy eating pattern.

Hydration also impacts metabolism and nutrient absorption. Proper hydration is necessary for the optimal functioning of the digestive system. Inadequate hydration can slow down the digestion process, potentially leading to discomfort and reduced nutrient absorption. By staying hydrated, individuals can ensure that their bodies efficiently process the nutrients from the foods they consume, enhancing the benefits of a balanced diet.

Furthermore, hydration can influence food choices. When we are dehydrated, we may experience a lack of energy and focus. This can lead to cravings for quick sources of energy, such as sugary snacks and caffeine. In contrast, being adequately hydrated supports cognitive function, concentration, and sustained energy levels. As a result, individuals are more likely to make thoughtful and health-conscious food choices that align with their nutritional goals.

Hydration is also closely linked to physical activity, which is an integral part of a healthy lifestyle. When we exercise, we lose fluids through sweat, and maintaining proper hydration levels becomes essential for performance and recovery. Dehydration can lead to decreased exercise performance, fatigue, and muscle cramps. To optimize physical activity and enhance the benefits of a balanced diet, it is crucial to stay hydrated before, during, and after exercise.

In conclusion, the relationship between hydration and healthy eating habits is multifaceted and impactful. Adequate hydration supports mindful eating, appetite regulation, portion control, metabolism, nutrient absorption, and cognitive function. By recognizing the importance of hydration, individuals can make more informed dietary choices, foster a deeper connection with their bodies, and ultimately improve their overall well-being. To promote healthy eating habits, it is imperative to prioritize hydration as an integral component of a holistic approach to health.

Chapter 6

Limit Process Meals

Limiting processed meals can greatly contribute to promoting a healthy diet. Processed meals, often high in added sugars, unhealthy fats, and sodium, can have detrimental effects on overall health. Here's a comprehensive overview of how reducing the consumption of processed meals can positively impact one's diet:

Nutrient Density: Whole, unprocessed foods like fruits, vegetables, whole grains, lean proteins, and nuts are rich in essential nutrients such as vitamins, minerals, fiber, and antioxidants. By consuming more of these foods and fewer processed meals, individuals can ensure they're getting a broader range of nutrients necessary for optimal health.

Reduced Added Sugars: Many processed meals contain hidden sugars, which can contribute to weight gain, insulin resistance, and other metabolic issues. By choosing whole foods, individuals can control their sugar intake and reduce the risk of developing conditions like type 2 diabetes.

Healthy Fats: Processed meals often contain unhealthy trans fats and excessive saturated fats. Opting for whole foods allows individuals to consume healthier fats, such as those found in avocados, nuts, seeds, and fatty fish, which can support heart health and overall well-being.

Lower Sodium Intake: Processed meals tend to be high in sodium, which can lead to hypertension and other cardiovascular problems. Preparing meals from scratch allows individuals to regulate their salt intake and make healthier choices for flavoring, like herbs and spices.

Fiber Content: Whole foods are generally higher in dietary fiber, which supports digestive health, helps control blood sugar levels, and promotes a feeling of fullness. Processed meals often lack sufficient fiber, contributing to overeating and digestive issues.

Control over Ingredients: Preparing meals at home provides control over ingredient quality and allows for customization based on personal dietary needs and preferences. This can be especially beneficial for individuals with allergies, intolerances, or specific nutritional goals.

Mindful Eating: Preparing meals from whole foods encourages mindfulness about food choices. This practice can help individuals become more attuned to their hunger and fullness cues, leading to better portion control and a healthier relationship with food.

Weight Management: Processed meals are often energy-dense and lack nutritional value, which can contribute to overconsumption of calories. Choosing whole, nutrient-dense foods can help manage weight by providing essential nutrients without excessive calories.

Long-Term Health Benefits: A diet rich in whole foods has been associated with a lower risk of chronic diseases such as heart disease, obesity, and certain types of cancer. Avoiding processed meals is a proactive step toward better long-term health.

Improved Energy Levels: The balanced nutrients found in whole foods can provide sustained energy throughout the day, whereas processed meals high in sugar and unhealthy fats can lead to energy crashes and fatigue.

Positive Impact on Mental Health: A well-balanced diet consisting of whole foods can positively affect mood and cognitive function. Nutrients like omega-3 fatty acids, B vitamins, and antioxidants support brain health and emotional well-being.

Culinary Skills: Preparing meals from scratch can foster an interest in cooking, leading to the development of valuable culinary skills and an appreciation for the art of cooking and creating nutritious meals.

In conclusion, limiting processed meals and prioritizing whole, unprocessed foods can have a significant impact on overall health and well-being. The nutrient density, reduced added sugars, healthy fats, lower sodium intake, and other benefits of consuming whole foods contribute to a healthier lifestyle, making it an essential practice for promoting optimal health.

Limit Late Night Meals

Limiting nighttime eating can indeed contribute to promoting healthy eating habits. Here's a comprehensive overview of how it can be beneficial:

Improved Digestion: Eating late at night can disrupt your body's natural circadian rhythm and digestive processes. Our metabolism tends to slow down in the evening, making it harder for our bodies to properly digest and process food.

Calorie Control: Nighttime eating often involves consuming extra calories that your body may not need for energy. By setting a cut-off time for eating, you reduce the likelihood of consuming unnecessary calories, helping to maintain a healthy weight.

Blood Sugar Regulation: Late-night snacking, especially on high-sugar or high-carbohydrate foods, can cause rapid spikes and crashes in blood sugar levels. These fluctuations can impact insulin sensitivity and increase the risk of type 2 diabetes. Limiting nighttime eating can help stabilize blood sugar levels and promote better metabolic health.

Mindful Eating: Establishing a firm eating window encourages mindful eating throughout the day. Knowing that you won't be eating late at night encourages you to make healthier choices earlier in the day, as you're less likely to "save" calories for a late-night snack.

Improved Sleep Quality: Late-night meals can disrupt sleep patterns and quality. Digestion requires energy, which can interfere with your body's ability to wind down and prepare for sleep. By avoiding heavy meals close to bedtime, you allow your body to rest more comfortably and improve sleep hygiene.

Enhanced Hydration: Nighttime eating can sometimes involve salty or processed foods, leading to water retention and dehydration. By avoiding these late-night snacks, you can better prioritize hydration and overall well-being.

Coping Mechanisms: Nighttime eating can sometimes be linked to emotional or stress-related eating. By setting boundaries on when you eat, you're more likely to identify and address emotional triggers, finding healthier ways to cope with stress or emotions.

Balanced Nutrition: Limiting nighttime eating encourages a more structured eating schedule, making it easier to plan balanced meals and snacks throughout the day. This can help ensure you're getting the right nutrients and fuel for your body's needs.

Intuitive Eating: Allowing your body to rest and rejuvenate during the evening and night supports the principles of intuitive eating. You learn to eat when you're truly hungry and honor your body's signals rather than eating out of habit or boredom.

Positive Habit Formation: Consistently avoiding nighttime eating can help you develop a strong habit of making healthier choices and adhering to a structured eating routine. Over time, this can lead to a more positive relationship with food and a greater sense of control over your eating patterns.

Remember, promoting healthy eating habits isn't solely about when you eat, but also about what you eat and how you approach food. Combining a balanced diet with mindful eating practices and a well-structured eating schedule can contribute to overall better health and well-being.

Having a Proper Meal Diet

Breakfast:

Oatmeal topped with sliced bananas, a handful of walnuts, and a drizzle of honey.

Whole-grain toast with avocado spread, a poached egg, and a side of berries.

Greek yogurt parfait with granola, mixed berries, and a sprinkle of chia seeds.

Lunch:

Grilled chicken or tempeh wrap with whole-wheat tortilla, mixed greens, tomatoes, cucumbers, and a light dressing.

Lentil and vegetable soup with a side salad of mixed greens, bell peppers, and a balsamic vinaigrette.

Quinoa salad with chickpeas, roasted red peppers, feta cheese, and a lemon-tahini dressing.

Snacks:

Cottage cheese with pineapple chunks and a small handful of almonds.

Apple slices with natural peanut butter.

Dinner:

Baked cod with roasted Brussels sprouts, quinoa, and a lemon-dill sauce.

Stir-fried tofu with broccoli, bell peppers, snap peas, and brown rice.

Grilled vegetable and black bean burrito bowl with salsa, guacamole, and a sprinkle of shredded cheese.

Dessert (occasional):

Dark chocolate dipped strawberries.

Greek yogurt with a drizzle of honey and chopped mixed nuts.

Beverages:

Water should be your primary choice throughout the day.

Tips:

whole grains such as brown rice, quinoa, whole-wheat pasta, Aim for a variety of colourful fruits and vegetables for a wide range of nutrients.

Include lean protein sources like poultry, fish, tofu, legumes, and nuts.

Opt for and whole-grain bread.

Use healthy fats like olive oil, avocados, nuts, and seeds in moderation.

Monitor portion sizes to avoid overeating.

Plan your meals and snacks ahead of time for better adherence to the healthy eating plan.

Remember, it's important to tailor your diet to your individual needs and consult a healthcare professional or registered dietitian for personalized guidance.

Chapter 7

Practice Intuitive Eating

Intuitive eating is an approach to food and eating that promotes healthy eating habits by focusing on your body's natural cues and instincts. Here's how it can promote healthy eating habits:

Listening to Your Body: Intuitive eating encourages you to pay attention to your body's hunger and fullness cues. This means eating when you're hungry and stopping when you're satisfied, which can help prevent overeating.

No Food Restrictions: It rejects strict diets and food rules. Allowing yourself to eat a wide variety of foods, including those you enjoy, reduces the allure of forbidden foods, reducing the likelihood of binge eating or unhealthy cravings.

Mindful Eating: Intuitive eating emphasizes mindfulness, which means being fully present while eating. This can help you savor your food, recognize when you're satisfied, and prevent overeating.

Respect for Your Body: It promotes body acceptance and respect. When you accept your body as it is, you're more likely to make choices that support its well-being, such as nourishing it with nutritious foods and engaging in physical activity you enjoy.

Emotional Eating: Intuitive eating addresses emotional eating by encouraging you to find alternative ways to cope with emotions rather than using food as a comfort. This can lead to better emotional well-being and healthier eating patterns.

Long-Term Approach: Unlike fad diets, intuitive eating is a sustainable, lifelong approach. It helps you build a positive relationship with food and your body, which can lead to lasting healthy eating habits.

Improved Body Image: By focusing on how your body feels and functions rather than just its appearance, intuitive eating can lead to improved body image. This can reduce the drive for extreme diets or unhealthy weight loss methods.

Reduced Stress: Letting go of food rules and restrictions can reduce the stress associated with dieting. Lower stress levels can indirectly promote healthier eating habits because stress can lead to emotional eating or cravings for unhealthy foods.

In summary, intuitive eating promotes healthy eating habits by encouraging a balanced, sustainable, and mindful approach to food and nutrition, while also fostering a positive relationship with your body and food choices.

Cultivating a Healthy Eating Habit

Snack Wisely

In today's fast-paced world, the concept of snacking has evolved significantly. Snacks are no longer just a treat or a quick energy fix; they have become an integral part of our daily diet. When done right, snacking can play a crucial role in promoting healthy eating habits. In this article, we will explore the importance of snacking properly and how it can contribute to a healthier lifestyle.

Understanding the Role of Snacking:

To comprehend the significance of snacking in promoting healthy eating habits, it's essential to first understand why we snack. Snacking serves several purposes, including:

Sustaining Energy Levels: Snacking can help maintain steady blood sugar levels throughout the day, preventing energy crashes that often lead to poor food choices later on.

Nutrient Intake: It provides an opportunity to incorporate essential nutrients like vitamins, minerals, and fiber into our diet. This is especially important for people with busy lifestyles who **may not always have time for full meals.**

Managing Hunger: Snacking can curb excessive hunger between meals, reducing the likelihood of overeating during main meals.

However, the key lies in snacking properly, which involves making mindful choices regarding both the types and timing of snacks.

Choosing the Right Snacks:

The types of snacks we choose can significantly impact our overall health. Opting for nutrient-dense snacks over empty-calorie options can make a substantial difference. Here are some guidelines for selecting healthier snack options:

Choose Whole Grains: Whole-grain snacks like whole-grain crackers, popcorn, or whole-grain granola bars provide complex carbohydrates and fiber, helping to keep you full and satisfied.

Include Lean Proteins: Snacks containing lean protein sources like Greek yogurt, nuts, or hummus with whole-grain crackers can help maintain muscle mass and promote satiety.

Minimize Processed Foods: Reduce the intake of highly processed and sugary snacks, such as candy, chips, and sugary drinks.

Hydrate Wisely: Water is a vital part of any diet. Sometimes,Stay hydrated throughout the day to avoid unnecessary snacking.

The Importance of Timing:

Beyond the types of snacks, the timing of your snacking matters too. The goal is to prevent excessive hunger and maintain energy levels without overloading on calories. Here are some timing tips for effective snacking:

Regular Intervals: Aim for snacks between meals at regular intervals. Snack when you're genuinely hungry rather than out of habit or boredom.

Pre-Workout and Post-Workout: Snacking before and after exercise can optimize your workout and recovery. A balanced snack with a mix of carbohydrates and protein can enhance performance and muscle repair.

Evening Snacks: If you tend to get hungry in the evening, choose a light and healthy snack to avoid overeating during dinner.

Snacking for Special Dietary Needs:

For individuals with specific dietary needs, such as those with diabetes, food allergies, or gluten intolerance, snacking properly becomes even more critical. It's essential to choose snacks that align with these dietary restrictions while still providing essential nutrients.

For example, individuals with diabetes should focus on snacks that help stabilize blood sugar levels, such as nuts, seeds, and vegetables with hummus. Those with gluten intolerance can opt for gluten-free whole-grain snacks like rice cakes or quinoa-based snacks.

Balancing Snacks with Meals:

While snacking can be beneficial, it's crucial to strike a balance with main meals. Snacks should complement, not replace, breakfast, lunch, and dinner. A well-balanced meal plan includes a combination of all food groups, ensuring you get a wide range of nutrients.

Incorporating lean proteins, whole grains, fruits, and vegetables into your meals alongside healthy snacks can provide a holistic approach to nutrition and promote a healthy eating habit.

The Psychological Aspect of Snacking:

Apart from the physical aspects, the psychology of snacking also plays a significant role in promoting healthy eating habits. Snacking can be a source of comfort, stress relief, or celebration. Recognizing and addressing emotional eating is crucial.

Emotional Awareness: When you feel the urge to snack due to emotions, consider alternative ways to cope, such as meditation, yoga, or talking to a friend.

Healthy Substitutions: If you have a craving for a specific snack, explore healthier alternatives. For example, if you crave something sweet, opt for a piece of dark chocolate instead of a high-sugar dessert.

In conclusion Snacking properly is a powerful tool in promoting healthy eating habits. By choosing nutrient-dense snacks, timing them strategically, and being mindful of your body's cues, you can enhance your overall nutrition and well-being. Remember that snacking is not a one-size-fits-all approach, and individual dietary needs and preferences should always be considered. When done thoughtfully, snacking can contribute to a balanced and sustainable approach to healthy eating, ultimately leading to better long-term health outcomes. So, the next time you reach for a snack, make it count towards a healthier you

Stress Management

In the world today stress has become a hindrance to healhty eating.The demands of work, family, and personal life can lead to chronic stress, which, in turn, can have a significant impact on our overall health. One area where stress can exert a particularly powerful influence is on our eating habits. Stress often leads to unhealthy eating patterns, but with effective stress management techniques, it is possible to promote and maintain healthy eating habits. In this article, we will explore the complex relationship between stress and nutrition, and how managing stress can contribute to better choices in our diet.

Stress and the Brain (The Craving Connection)

To understand how stress management can promote healthy eating habits, it's crucial to comprehend the intricate relationship between stress, the brain, and our dietary choices. When we experience stress, our brain triggers a cascade of hormonal responses, including the release of cortisol, often referred to as the "stress hormone." Cortisol influences various brain regions, including those involved in reward and motivation.

One of the consequences of elevated cortisol levels is an increase in cravings for high-calorie, high-sugar, and high-fat foods. These comfort foods provide a temporary sense of pleasure and relief from stress, leading individuals to indulge in them as a form of self-soothing. However, these foods are often nutritionally poor and can contribute to weight gain and various health issues when consumed regularly.

Moreover, stress can disrupt our normal eating patterns. Some people may lose their appetite when stressed, while others may turn to food for comfort. This behavior can create a vicious cycle where stress leads to poor dietary choices, which can, in turn, lead to weight gain and further exacerbate stress levels.

The Role of Stress Management

Effective stress management techniques can break this cycle and promote healthier eating habits. Here's how:

Stress Awareness: The first step in managing stress is recognizing it. By being aware of the stressors in your life and how they affect your eating habits, you can begin to take control of the situation. Mindfulness practices, such as meditation and journaling, can help increase awareness of stress triggers.

Stress Reduction: Engaging in stress-reduction activities can help lower cortisol levels and reduce the desire for unhealthy comfort foods. Exercise, yoga, and deep breathing techniques are effective ways to manage stress and improve mood, making it less likely to turn to food for emotional relief.

Healthy Coping Mechanisms: Rather than resorting to unhealthy foods to cope with stress, individuals can adopt healthier alternatives. Engaging in hobbies, spending time with loved ones, or seeking professional support through therapy are productive ways to deal with stress without resorting to emotional eating.

Meal Planning: Stress often leads to haphazard eating habits, such as skipping meals or choosing fast food for convenience. Planning meals in advance ensures that nutritious options are readily available, reducing the temptation to grab unhealthy snacks when stressed.

Nutrition Education: Learning about the nutritional value of foods can help individuals make informed choices even when stressed. Understanding the benefits of a balanced diet can provide motivation to opt for healthier options, even in stressful situations.

Social Support: Sharing your stress management and healthy eating goals with friends or family can provide accountability and encouragement. Social support can be a powerful motivator in making positive changes.

The Long-Term Benefits

The impact of stress management on promoting healthy eating habits extends beyond the immediate reduction in comfort eating. Over time, consistently making healthier food choices can lead to a range of long-term benefits:

Weight Management: Managing stress and making healthier food choices can contribute to weight loss or maintenance, reducing the risk of obesity-related health issues.

Improved Mood: A balanced diet can positively influence mood and mental well-being. Reduced stress and improved nutrition often go hand in hand, leading to a happier and more balanced life.

Better Physical Health: A nutritious diet supports overall physical health by providing essential nutrients, reducing the risk of chronic diseases like diabetes, heart disease, and certain cancers.

Enhanced Productivity: Lower stress levels and better nutrition can improve cognitive function and productivity, making it easier to manage daily responsibilities.

In conclusion, the relationship between stress and eating habits is complex but manageable. By implementing effective stress management techniques and prioritizing healthy coping mechanisms, individuals can break the cycle of stress-induced unhealthy eating. This, in turn, can lead to a cascade of positive long-term effects on physical and mental health. Stress management is not only about alleviating immediate discomfort; it's a pathway to a healthier, happier life through better nutrition and well-being.

Cultivating a Healthy Eating Habit

Stay Informed

However, one powerful tool that often goes overlooked in the quest for better nutrition is information. Staying informed about nutrition and food-related topics can be a game-changer in promoting healthy eating habits. In this word exploration, we will delve into the ways in which staying informed can contribute to a healthier lifestyle.

Understanding Nutritional Basics

One of the most obvious ways in which staying informed aids healthy eating habits is by providing a foundational understanding of nutrition. Knowledge about macronutrients (carbohydrates, proteins, and fats), micronutrients (vitamins and minerals), and their roles in the body allows individuals to make informed choices about what they consume. For example, knowing that fruits and vegetables are rich in essential vitamins and minerals encourages people to include them in their diets regularly.

Furthermore, understanding the basics of calories and portion control can help individuals maintain a healthy weight. Armed with information about calorie content, individuals can make conscious decisions about portion sizes and overall calorie intake. This knowledge can prevent overeating and contribute to weight management, a crucial aspect of long-term health.

Recognizing Food Labels

Food packaging can be a minefield of information, but it's also a valuable resource for those seeking to make healthy choices. Staying informed about how to read food labels empowers individuals to decipher the nutritional content of packaged foods. By examining labels for key information such as serving sizes, calorie counts, and the presence of additives or preservatives, consumers can make more informed decisions about the products they select.

Furthermore, staying informed about labeling regulations and health claims can help individuals avoid falling for marketing tricks. For example, understanding the difference between "low fat" and "low sugar" claims can prevent someone from choosing a product that seems healthy but is, in reality, laden with sugar. Knowledge is a shield against deceptive marketing tactics.

The world of nutrition is constantly evolving, with new dietary trends and fads emerging regularly. Staying informed about these trends is essential to navigate the ever-changing landscape of healthy eating. It enables individuals to separate evidence-based dietary advice from fleeting trends that may not provide long-term health benefits.

For instance, the keto diet gained immense popularity in recent years. Those who were well-informed could assess the diet's potential benefits and drawbacks, ensuring it aligned with their personal health goals. Staying informed also helps individuals understand when a particular trend might not be suitable for their specific needs or health conditions.

Addressing Dietary Restrictions and Allergies

Many individuals have dietary restrictions or allergies that require careful attention to their food choices. Staying informed about various dietary needs, such as gluten-free, dairy-free, or nut-free diets, is crucial for those affected and for those who prepare meals for them. Knowledge about safe ingredient substitutions and where to find suitable products can make a significant difference in the quality of life for individuals with dietary restrictions.

Promoting Healthy Eating in Communities

Beyond personal benefits, staying informed about nutrition can have a ripple effect on communities. When individuals prioritize healthy eating, they often become advocates for change in their social circles. They share knowledge, recipes, and resources, fostering a culture of health-consciousness that can positively influence the eating habits of friends and family.

Additionally, staying informed about local food systems and sustainable agriculture can encourage individuals to support local farmers and make eco-friendly food choices. These actions not only promote personal health but also contribute to the well-being of the environment and the community as a whole.

In conclusion, staying informed is a potent tool in the promotion of healthy eating habits. It equips individuals with the knowledge needed to make informed food choices, read labels accurately, navigate dietary trends wisely, address dietary restrictions, and advocate for healthy eating within their communities. In an era when convenience often overshadows nutrition, information serves as a beacon, guiding individuals towards better health. It empowers them to take control of their diets, make choices aligned with their well-being, and ultimately enjoy the benefits of a healthier lifestyle.

Limit Excessive Salt intake

Excessive salt consumption has been linked to various health issues, including high blood pressure, cardiovascular diseases, and kidney problems. By adopting strategies to limit salt intake, individuals can take significant steps towards promoting healthier eating habits and improving their overall quality of life

Understanding the Role of Salt:

Salt, composed of sodium and chloride, plays a vital role in our bodies, aiding in fluid balance, nerve transmission, and muscle function. However, the modern diet often contains an excess of salt, mainly due to processed and packaged foods. This surplus can lead to health problems, making it essential to adopt measures that promote moderation.

Reading Food Labels:

A fundamental step in reducing salt intake is to become a savvy food label reader. Food packaging provides information on sodium content per serving, allowing consumers to make informed choices. Opt for products with lower sodium levels and be mindful of serving sizes, as they can impact your overall sodium intake.

Cooking at Home:

Cooking meals at home empowers individuals to control the amount of salt used in their dishes. Experimenting with herbs, spices, and citrus flavors can enhance taste without relying on excessive salt. Gradually reducing the amount of salt used during cooking can help taste buds adjust to less salty flavors.

Choosing Fresh Ingredients:

Whole, unprocessed foods generally contain lower amounts of sodium compared to their processed counterparts. Fresh fruits, vegetables, lean proteins, and whole grains should form the core of a low-sodium diet. This approach not only limits salt intake but also provides essential nutrients that contribute to better health.

Limiting Processed Foods:

Processed foods, such as canned soups, snacks, and ready-to-eat meals, often contain hidden sodium. These items are convenient but can be laden with excessive salt. Whenever possible, opt for homemade alternatives or select products labeled as low-sodium or sodium-free.

Be Mindful at Restaurants:

Eating out can be enjoyable, but restaurant meals tend to be high in salt due to flavor enhancement. Choose dishes with fewer sauces or dressings, ask for sauces on the side, and request that your meal be prepared with minimal salt. Being assertive about your preferences can significantly impact your salt intake.

Gradual Reduction Approach:

Abruptly cutting out salt from your diet may lead to dissatisfaction with taste. Instead, adopt a gradual reduction approach. Over time, your taste buds will adapt to lower salt levels, and you'll find yourself craving less salt.

Hydration and Water Intake:

Staying hydrated can help flush out excess sodium from the body. Drinking enough water supports overall health and can aid in reducing the negative effects of high salt consumption.

Awareness of Hidden Sodium:

Some foods that don't taste salty may still contain substantial sodium levels. Breads, cheeses, and even breakfast cereals can contribute to daily sodium intake. Being aware of these hidden sources allows for better planning and smarter choices.

Meal Planning and Preparation:

Planning meals ahead of time gives you control over ingredients and portion sizes. This approach reduces the likelihood of resorting to high-sodium convenience foods when hunger strikes.

Community Support and Accountability:

Embarking on a journey to limit salt intake is often more successful when done with a support system. Engage friends, family, or online communities that share similar goals. Sharing experiences, recipes, and tips can keep motivation high.

Consulting a Healthcare Professional:

If you have existing health conditions or concerns, consulting a healthcare professional or registered dietitian is advisable.

In conclusion, adopting a diet with limited salt intake is a vital step towards promoting healthy eating habits. By reading labels, cooking at home, choosing fresh ingredients, and being mindful of hidden sources of sodium, individuals can reduce their risk of health complications associated with excessive salt consumption. Remember that the journey to healthier eating is a gradual process, and with dedication and persistence, one can achieve a balanced and flavorful diet that supports long-term well-being

www.ingramcontent.com/pod-product-compliance
Lightning Source LLC
Chambersburg PA
CBHW071604270726
48661CB00018B/1245